Contents

What is MCT Oil?..4

Components of MCT oil...7

The Health and Fitness Benefits of MCT Oil..........9

    Fitness benefits of MCT oil....................................9

    Health benefits of MCT oil...................................10

    Controls Obesity:...11

    Increases Energy Levels:.......................................11

    Immune System:..12

    Improves Digestion:..12

    Boosts Heart Health:...13

    Maintains Hormone Balance:...............................13

    Prevents Diabetes:...13

    Improves Cognitive Function:..............................14

    Neuroprotective Benefits:....................................14

7 Health Benefits..16

    1. Weight Loss...16

    2. Brain Fuel..17

3. Reduce Lactate Accumulation 18

4. Manage Epilepsy, Alzheimer's Disease and Autism 19

5. Antimicrobial and Antifungal Properties 19

6. Reduce Risk for Heart Disease 20

7. Control Blood Sugar and Aid in Management of Diabetes 20

Ways to Use MCT Oil 21

How to use MCT Oil 22

Where to Get MCT Oil 23

What Are the Best MCT Oil Brands? 25

MCT Oil: A Potential Alzheimer's Treatment 27

Prescription MCT Oil for Alzheimer's Patients 28

Risks Associated with MCT Oil 29

Inflammation – 30

Digestion – 30

Anxiety – 31

Appetite – 31

Type 1 Diabetes – 32

Other Side Effects 32

MCT Oil Dosage 33

Major Facts about MCT Oils 34

Ways to keep your brain young 41

Popular Uses for MCT Oil 46

How MCT Oil Fuels the Brain 48

MCT Oil: A Buyers Guide 49

Conclusion 55

What is MCT Oil?

MCT oil is a medium-chain triglyceride that contains medium-length chains of fats called triglycerides, which due to their shorter lengths, are easier to digest.

MCT oil is commonly extracted from coconut oil, since nearly half of its contents contain MCTs.

They are widely known as beneficial nutrients for the body. These are commonly considered "good" forms of fat, which can do everything from boost the metabolism to improve the strength of the immune system. These medium-chain fatty acids (MCFA or MCT oils) are named C-6 (caproic acid), C-8 (caprylic acid), C-10 (capric acid) and C-12 (lauric acid). All of these acids are also found in coconut oil, which is why many people confuse the two. However, the majority of medium-chain fatty acids found in coconut oil (a total of 50-65% of the fats) are lauric acid.

The numbers attached to these fatty acids are important; the smaller ones (caproic, caprylic and capric acids) are easier for the body to absorb and convert directly into ketones, a powerful form of energy for the body. Lauric acid (C-12) is right on the edge of medium-chain fatty acids (6-12 carbons) and long-chain fatty acids (13 -21 carbons), and in some ways, it behaves like a long-chain fatty acid. It is slightly less efficiently processed by the body into energy but is still considered an MCT.

MCT oil is composed solely of these medium-chain fatty acids (100% versus the 50-65% in coconut oil). In this way, MCT oil is a more concentrated form of one or more of these beneficial fatty acids, some of which are rarer than others.

This is not to say that coconut oil does not have an impressive list of proven health benefits, but for those people who want an even stronger dose of antioxidant, anti-inflammatory and immune-boosting fatty acids, some type of MCT oil is the right choice. Again, some MCT oils will be a blend of these fatty acids, while other MCT oil products on the market will be 100% pure versions of one of these triglycerides. It is important to take note of these concentrations before adding this oil to your daily or weekly health regimen.

Components of MCT oil

C-6 (Caproic Acid): This is a medium-chain fatty acid that is in extremely small concentrations in most MCT oils, and is often processed out of them intentionally. It has a rather unpleasant taste, but as with other MCTs, it can be quickly converted into useful ketones and ATP, valuable "clean" energy sources in the body.

C-8 (Caprylic Acid): This is arguably the most important medium-chain fatty acid, but it is found in low concentrations in coconut oil. It is converted extremely quickly into ATP – usable energy – without involving the liver and is directly linked to improved cognition. It also results in a burst of energy and provides immune system support, thanks to its antioxidant and antibacterial qualities.

C-10 (Capric Acid): Another relatively rare MCT in coconut oil, this fatty acid is another type of fat that can bypass any lengthy processing in the liver, like a long-chain carbohydrate, such as a sugar. This makes capric acid ideal for rapidly producing energy within the body.

C-12 (Lauric Acid): With a 12-carbon chain, lauric acid does need to pass through the liver to be processed into energy, which makes it more like long-chain fatty acids. That being said, lauric acid also has antimicrobial properties, but it has a larger impact on your cholesterol than the smaller-chain MCTs.

The Health and Fitness Benefits of MCT Oil

Fitness benefits of MCT oil

Most of the health benefits surrounding the MCT oil hype have to do with weight loss and your metabolism, and one study found that people saw more weight loss and decreased body fat from consuming MCT oil rather than olive oil. The weight-loss bonus MCT oil provides could have much to do with the higher burn rate, meaning your body is able to quickly metabolize the fat, giving your metabolism a little boost in the process.

Research has also looked at whether MCT oil could be used to treat certain GI conditions related to the malabsorption of nutrients. It's the "rapid and simple" digestion of MCTs that might be the key, reports one paper published in Practical Gastroenterology. Turns out, the length of a fatty-acid chain influences its digestion and absorption within the GI tract. Some people cannot digest longer chains efficiently and therefore don't get the nutrients the body needs, but they are able to successfully digest and absorb these fast-metabolizing MCTs.

Other studies also link MCTs to decreased cardiovascular disease and Alzheimer's, "but that research is very limited," says Crandall.

But here's the interesting thing that's separating MCT oil from the pack. "None of the benefits of MCT oil have been shown to be true with coconut oil," says Crandall. Why not? Again, it all comes down to the kind of saturated fat found in those medium chains.

Health benefits of MCT oil

Using MCT oil is very effective for people who struggle with low energy, poor digestive health, obesity, hormonal fluctuations, slow metabolism, dementia, diabetes and inflammatory conditions, as well as those who are at high risk for cardiovascular disease.

Controls Obesity:

When the fatty acids of MCT oil are converted into energy, the metabolism is inevitably sped up, which can help with passive fat-burning and general efficiency of calorie burning by the body. In fact, research has shown that MCTs will prevent fat deposition by the body, instead of becoming pure forms of energy.

Increases Energy Levels:

With a boosted metabolism, you also have enhanced energy levels, not to mention the direct stream of ATP and ketones from the rapid conversion of MCTs to energy. Instead of more than 20 steps that sugar takes to become energy, C-8 medium-chain fatty acids can be converted to usable energy in only 3 steps, giving your body rapid support and invigorating you.

Immune System:

The antimicrobial qualities of lauric acid and caprylic acid make MCT oil a worthy immune system supporter, and there has been plenty of research on linking these to better overall health. There is an increase in immune activity and white blood cell production in the body, while the antioxidant effects of these acids also reduce levels of oxidative stress.

Improves Digestion:

Aside from its laxative qualities, MCT oil also has anti-inflammatory, antiviral and antibacterial qualities that can optimize digestion and balance the micro-environment of your gut flora. This will help prevent symptoms of cramping, bloating and constipation, as well as any parasitic or viral infections.

Boosts Heart Health:

One of the main factors leading to cardiovascular disease and heart problems is obesity, and with the low-fat deposition effect of MCT oil, there is a better chance of remaining slim, keeping overall cholesterol levels down, and lower blood pressure. While consuming fats may seem counterintuitive to heart health, most MCTs are those "good" fats you need in your diet.

Maintains Hormone Balance:

One of the critical purposes of fats in the body is their role in creating hormones. With these MCTs in your diet, you can make those hormones you need most to keep your mood in place, your metabolism high, and prevent depression and hormonal disorders.

Prevents Diabetes:

MCTs are known to help control blood sugar, namely by preventing fat deposition, and instead of storing sugars in muscle and energy sources. Given that MCT oil can help control obesity, increase the metabolism and optimize digestion, this oil is not only good for people with diabetes but also those at high risk of the disease.

Improves Cognitive Function:

When small medium-chain fatty acids convert directly into ketones, one of the areas where these are believed to have the most effect is in the brain. By providing energy to and protecting neural pathways, these ketones can mitigate the symptoms of dementia and other neurodegenerative diseases, by providing energy for concentration, focus and memory retention.

Here are some of its benefits to the brain

Neuroprotective Benefits:

MCTs offer neuroprotective benefits for a wide range of diseases including dementia,

Alzheimer's, Parkinson's, stroke, epilepsy, and traumatic brain injury.

Delay Brain Aging: MCTs can delay brain aging by providing extra fuel to repair brain cell damage, especially when combined with a high-fat diet.

Depression and Autism: Caprylic acid, a main component of MCT oil supplements, holds promise for treating autism and depression.

Increase Brain Energy: Taking MCT oil has been found to increase brain energy by 8 to 9%.

Optimize Intestinal Flora: MCT oil can help optimize your intestinal flora surprisingly important to brain health. Among other things, good bacteria produce dozens of neurotransmitters, including more than 90% of your total serotonin and 50% of your dopamine.

7 Health Benefits

1. Weight Loss

There are several ways in which MCT oil promotes weight loss, one of which is the production of two hormones that make you feel fuller: peptide YY and leptin.

A study found that taking 2 tablespoons MCT oil at breakfast kept participants fuller into lunchtime when compared to just taking coconut oil.

MCT oil can reduce your waist line due to in part because it contains 10% less calories than long-chain triglycerides (LCTs), found in olive oil, nuts and avocados.

And since MCT oil is easier to digest, it can promote weight loss in a couple of ways.

The body doesn't store MCTs as body fat because it can be readily used as an energy source.

Think of shorter-chain triglycerides as your body not having to undergo as many steps in the break-down process compared to longer chains.

The great thing about MCT oil, specifically for keto dieting, is that it can be converted to ketones when the body's in a low carb state, keeping you in fat-burning ketosis.

Another advantage of MCT oil is that it's great for gut health.

Gut health, in turn, supports healthy gut fauna (good probiotic bacteria) that supports weight loss.

2. Brain Fuel

Aside from the multitude of ways MCT oil powers weight loss, let's talk about how it can be used as a major source of brain fuel.

We've already discussed how MCT oil is rapidly absorbed by the body due to its short length.

MCTs doesn't require the need for bile to break it down, altogether skipping this lengthy process.

Instead it goes straight to the liver where it can be used instantly by cells.

The liver is also where MCTs are converted into ketones.

Ketones act as a fuel for your brain since they can readily pass through the blood-brain barrier.

3. Reduce Lactate Accumulation

During exercise, lactate levels rise due to biochemical processes in muscle cells.

Lactate acid is what causes soreness after an intense workout and can lead to a loss of productivity as there's often too much discomfort to continue exercise.

This is where MCT oil comes to play.

A study found that by taking 1.5 teaspoons MCT oil before exercise, you can lower lactate levels.

The same study found that MCT oil can also help you burn fat instead of carbs, which is crucial for those wanting to lose weight more effectively.

4. Manage Epilepsy, Alzheimer's Disease and Autism

Ketones have been shown to reduce epileptic seizures, act as a brain energy source for Alzheimer's patients, and manage autism.

Note: If you intend to use MCT oil to manage these conditions, be sure to talk to a doctor first to evaluate the risks and advantanges.

5. Antimicrobial and Antifungal Properties

Coconut oil has been shown to reduce both bacterial and yeast growth in the lab.

However, more human studies need to be done to properly evaluate its effects.

6. Reduce Risk for Heart Disease

MCTs support weight loss which in turn reduces your risk for heart disease.

Adding MCT oil into your diet can lower your levels of LDL, or "low-density lipoproteins", and increase your levels of HDL ("high-density lipoproteins").

In addition, MCT oil has been shown to significantly reduce C-reactive protein (CRP) that's released due to inflammation and increases your risk of heart disease.

7. Control Blood Sugar and Aid in Management of Diabetes

MCT oil can also help control blood sugar in people with diabetes.

Ways to Use MCT Oil

MCT oil is a lightly flavored oil you can add to any low-heat recipe (high heat will render it off).

Add it to smoothies, salad dressings, and coffee for a fatty supplement.

Other options include oatmeal, yogurt, protein shakes, and homemade ice cream.

In conclusion, MCT oil can be a great tool for anyone on the keto diet, though it's not something to be taken in excess.

How to use MCT Oil

MCT oil is available as both a liquid and as a powder supplement.

You can take the oil by the spoonful or mix the powder with any drink.

Since it is virtually tasteless, the uses for MCT oil are limited only by your imagination.

Medium-chain triglycerides are water soluble and so MCT oil readily mixes with foods.

You can add it to smoothies, soups, stews, yogurt, salad dressings, spreads, and drinks of all kinds, both hot and cold.

But don't cook with it since it has a low smoke point and burns at 150° C (302° F).

Where to Get MCT Oil

Supplement retailers and health food grocers market moderately priced MCT oil and powder for $14 to $30. But Crandall notes that these oils are all "proprietary blends" that, like coconut oil, only contain some MCT and won't be the exact ratio of palm and coconut MCTs used in labs and research. This "medical-grade" MCT oil mixture isn't available to the public, but Crandall estimates that if it were, it would cost you more like $200 for a tiny 8-oz container. So for now, you'll have to read ingredient labels and work with what you've got.

Currently, there are no guidelines or regulations on whether a proprietary blend can label a product "pure, 100% MCT oil." "These brands do not have to divulge what their blends are, and there are no official supplement standards that must be met," she says.

So how do you know if the MCT oil or supplement you find on the shelf is legit? Crandall calls this the "lab-rat stage." While everyone's digestive system is different, she suggests finding an MCT oil that is a mix of coconut and palm oils (avoid anything that says it's simply a coconut derivative), and then start small and see how your body reacts. Below are the places you can get MCT oil

MCT Online Retailers

Amazon

Jet.com

EVitamins

The best place to purchase MCT oil is from your local health food store. You can find one or more options at the following locations:

What Are the Best MCT Oil Brands?

To avoid MCT oil products that may contain harmful solvents and unnecessary ingredients, you want to be sure to avoid purchasing low-quality products. Consumers consistently rank the following MCT oil brands the highest.

BulletProof Brain Octane

NOW Foods MCT Oil

Onnit MCT Oil

NuMedica MCT Oil USP

Bulletproof XCT Oil

Viva Labs MCT Oil

Sports Research MCT Oil

Swanson Premium 100% Pure MCT Oil

Caveman Coffee Co MCT Oil

Twinlab MCT Fuel

Try MCT Oil

MCT Oil: A Potential Alzheimer's Treatment

One of the most promising uses for MCT oil is in treating dementia and Alzheimer's.

Alzheimer's is believed to be a type of diabetes of the brain caused by brain cells losing their ability to absorb glucose, their main source of energy, which leads to their death.

PET scans show that areas of the brain affected by Alzheimer's readily take up ketones as an alternative fuel source. While ketogenic diets can be useful for dementia and Alzheimer's patients, it is notoriously difficult to get them to change their eating habits.

Prescription MCT Oil for Alzheimer's Patients

Alzheimer's patients and their caretakers may understandably be concerned about the use of any supplement that hasn't been doctor-recommended.

In that case, talk to your doctor about the prescription-only "medical food" called Axona which contains a proprietary formulation of medium-chain triglycerides.

It was created to help manage mild to moderate symptoms of Alzheimer's disease.

Risks Associated with MCT Oil

There are a number of potential side effects of using MCT oil, including hormone fluctuations, gastrointestinal distress, anxiety, appetite abnormality, headaches and inflammation, and can also negatively affect people with certain liver conditions or diabetes. You are particularly susceptible to these side effects if you use the oil in too high of a dose. The concentration of medium-chain fatty acids in MCT oil is enough to quickly remedy most afflictions. Always speak to your doctor about using this oil with your particular condition, and discontinue use if serious negative side effects occur.

Hormones –

When the medium-chain fatty acids are processed by the body, it happens quickly, which tends to generate heat and energy. This can stimulate the metabolism and cause hormone fluctuations in certain people, as well as hot flashes. There may be mild irritability or mood swings, particularly if you are taking too much of the oil.

Inflammation –

Your body receives a burst of pure and positive energy from the processing of certain true medium-chain triglycerides. This can be a bit overwhelming for your system, if not taken in moderation, which can temporarily increase your blood pressure and cause inflammation or headaches. Consider lessening your dosage if this occurs. Throat itchiness and respiratory irritation can also occur.

Digestion –

These medium-chain triglycerides are known to stimulate the stomach, and have laxative effects due to their powerful impact on digestion. Excessive consumption of MCT oil can cause diarrhea, nausea, vomiting, flatulence and general stomach discomfort.

Anxiety –

While uncommon, some people report increased feelings of anxiety after consuming large amounts of MCT oil. This could be due to the rapid energy surge in your body, and without any way to expend that energy, it can manifest as anxiety or nervousness.

Appetite –

MCT oil has been known to cause both a loss of appetite and extreme hunger, although the latter is far less common. In terms of the former, the valuable energy produced by the acids makes the body feel as though it is full, which causes a decrease in appetite.

Liver Health – As mentioned, caprylic, caproic and capric acids all bypass the liver when being converted into energy, but that isn't true for lauric acid. It must be processed by the liver, so if you have existing liver problems, it is best to speak with a doctor before using MCT oil. While some MCT oils eliminate lauric acid (C-12), not all of them do.

Type 1 Diabetes –

Certain aspects of MCTs can help with diabetes, but if you have too many ketones in the body, those will be exclusively used for energy production, meaning that the body will continue to store up glucose until it is at a dangerous level. Speak to your doctor before using MCT oil if you have Type 1 diabetes.

Other Side Effects

There are few risks that come with using MCT oil, but two main drawbacks to consider are

1. MCT oil can initiate hunger hormones in some people and

2. can lead to fatty liver if taken in abundance.

With that in mind, MCT oil should only be taken as part of your total fat intake, not as a supplement since it is very high in calories.

MCT Oil Dosage

In terms of dosage, MCT oil usage will be different for everyone, depending on their personal health and wellness goals. However, to have an effect on most health conditions, no more than 2-3 tablespoons per day are ever needed. In fact, that amount is on the high end. Most people find 1-2 teaspoons per day can help certain conditions, but everyone is different. The average range is between 2 teaspoons and 2 tablespoons per day.

Major Facts about MCT Oils

IMPORTANT FACT 1

MCTs burn fat and are a sugar and caffeine free way to increase energy naturally.

Simply put, MCT oil is certain types of healthy fats in an oil form. What makes MCTs so special are their molecular makeup. Fat molecules include a "body" and a "tail" of a chain of carbon and hydrogen molecules that vary in length.

MCT stands for Medium-Chain Triglycerides, which are in between the longer and shorter chain fat molecules.

MCTs have been found to be easiest for the body to break down and use as a naturally produced energy source without the storage of excess fat in the body or any of the "crashing" effects of sugar or caffeine.

MCT oil is virtually clear, odorless, and tasteless oil that can be added to drinks, dressings, and more!

IMPORTANT FACT 2

MCT oils are not all created equal. There are only 2 considered true and are the most effective for fueling energy without slowing your metabolism.

There are many different types of MCT oils but the 2 most effective for a quick energy source without slowing down your metabolism are called C8 (Caprylic Acid) and C10 (Capric Acid) – they are so called for the number of carbons molecules in their chain. These 2 types of MCT oil are considered "true biological" MCT oils and are the only two to bypass the liver process and convert directly into energy.

C8 (Caprylic Acid) can help maintain a healthy gut and is the fastest to metabolize in the brain, and C10 (Capric Acid) is it is the second shortest chain to quickly bypass the liver and be converted directly into energy.

The Ketogenic diet has really brought MCT oil into the spotlight recently as being one of the top recommended ketogenic supplements to use when following the diet plan. This is mainly because adding MCTs to your diet can increase the number of carbs you can eat while remaining in fat burning state of ketosis.

IMPORTANT FACT 3

KETO & PALEO folks love it, but MCT oil has amazing health benefits for all!

Even if you are not following a Ketogenic diet plan, MCT oil can be used for some great health benefits such as weight management, increased energy and cognitive focus, and cardiovascular and gut health.

MCTs have been shown to improve mental performance

MCTs can provide a natural source of energy for the brain and muscles

MCTs are not stimulants-they do not raise heart rate or blood pressure

Studies show that MCTs (mainly C8 and C10) may increase the body's ability to burn fat and calories

Studies found that MCTs balance hormones that help reduce appetite and help increase feelings of fullness

MCTs support digestion and nutrient absorption

IMPORTANT FACT 4

To experience maximum health benefits a high quality organic MCT oil from the best source is a must!

You can get trace amounts of MCT oils from foods directly but most of the time there is not enough true MCTs for the maximum benefits. For the most effective, concentrated amount of MCTs 8 and 10, a high quality, properly sourced, 100% organic MCT oil is the way to go.

Perfect MCT Oil: 100%

Coconut oil: 15% (Mostly other types of MCTs that have other health benefits)

Palm kernel oil: 7.9% (highly recommended to not use)

Cheese: 7.3% (not a high source)

Butter: 6.8% (not a high source)

Milk: 6.9% (not a high source)

Yogurt: 6.6% (not a high source

IMPORTANT FACT 5

NEVER use Palm kernel based MCT oil!

The palm oil industry is responsible for the deforestation for large parts of the rainforest and the large-scale production of palm crops in these areas are driving native people from their homes. It is highly recommended to use MCT oils derived from coconut oil, which is more environmentally conscious and sustainable.

Ways to keep your brain young

1. Get mental stimulation

Through research with mice and humans, scientists have found that brainy activities stimulate new connections between nerve cells and may even help the brain generate new cells, developing neurological "plasticity" and building up a functional reserve that provides a hedge against future cell loss.

Any mentally stimulating activity should help to build up your brain. Read, take courses, try "mental gymnastics," such as word puzzles or math problems Experiment with things that require manual dexterity as well as mental effort, such as drawing, painting, and other crafts.

2. Get physical exercise

Research shows that using your muscles also helps your mind. Animals who exercise regularly increase the number of tiny blood vessels that bring oxygen-rich blood to the region of the brain that is responsible for thought. Exercise also spurs the development of new nerve cells and increases the connections between brain cells (synapses). This results in brains that are more efficient, plastic, and adaptive, which translates into better performance in aging animals. Exercise also lowers blood pressure, improves cholesterol levels, helps blood sugar balance and reduces mental stress, all of which can help your brain as well as your heart.

3. Improve your diet

Good nutrition can help your mind as well as your body. For example, people that eat a Mediterranean style diet that emphasizes fruits, vegetables, fish, nuts, unsaturated oils (olive oil) and plant sources of proteins are less likely to develop cognitive impairment and dementia.

4. Improve your blood pressure

High blood pressure in midlife increases the risk of cognitive decline in old age. Use lifestyle modification to keep your pressure as low as possible. Stay lean, exercise regularly, limit your alcohol to two drinks a day, reduce stress, and eat right.

5. Improve your blood sugar

Diabetes is an important risk factor for dementia. You can help prevent diabetes by eating right, exercising regularly, and staying lean. But if your blood sugar stays high, you'll need medication to achieve good control.

6. Improve your cholesterol

High levels of LDL ("bad") cholesterol are associated with an increased the risk of dementia. Diet, exercise, weight control, and avoiding tobacco will go a long way toward improving your cholesterol levels. But if you need more help, ask your doctor about medication.

7. Consider low-dose aspirin

Some observational studies suggest that low-dose aspirin may reduce the risk of dementia, especially vascular dementia. Ask your doctor if you are a candidate.

8. Avoid tobacco

Avoid tobacco in all its forms.

9. Don't abuse alcohol

Excessive drinking is a major risk factor for dementia. If you choose to drink, limit yourself to two drinks a day.

10. Care for your emotions

People who are anxious, depressed, sleep-deprived, or exhausted tend to score poorly on cognitive function tests. Poor scores don't necessarily predict an increased risk of cognitive decline in old age, but good mental health and restful sleep are certainly important goals.

11. Protect your head

Moderate to severe head injuries, even without diagnosed concussions, increase the risk of cognitive impairment.

12. Build social networks

Strong social ties have been associated with a lower risk of dementia, as well as lower blood pressure and longer life expectancy.

Get the information you need to strengthen your intellectual prowess, promote your powers of recall, and protect the brain-based skills when you buy A Guide to Cognitive Fitness, a special health report by the experts at Harvard.

Popular Uses for MCT Oil

MCT oil is mostly sold as a supplement to aid weight loss or improve athletic performance.

It's popular with bodybuilders and endurance athletes who use it to increase energy and decrease body fat while increasing lean muscle mass.

But the scientific evidence to support these benefits of MCT oil is mixed.

And taking enough MCT oil to reap these benefits is not always practical.

For example, it's thought that to experience any significant weight loss, you'd have to eat half your daily calories in MCT oil.

And taking MCT oil for physical performance presents a dilemma since the amount of MCT oil needed to increase endurance generally is more than enough to cause diarrhea.

However, one area where MCT oil shows great promise is as a supplement to support brain health and function.

How MCT Oil Fuels the Brain

Your brain cannot store energy and so needs a constant stream that's usually supplied by blood glucose.

But there's a backup system for times your blood sugar gets low.

When needed, your liver can break down stored body fat to produce ketones.

Ketones readily cross the blood-brain barrier to provide instant energy to the brain.

And while you can provide ketones for your brain by eating a very high-fat, low-carbohydrate ketogenic diet, you don't have to.

The medium-chain fats in MCT oil (and its source, coconut oil) raise the blood level of ketones, providing a convenient workaround.

MCT Oil: A Buyers Guide

MCT oil is a supplement that has a variety of health benefits. MCTs – which stands for Medium Chain Triglycerides, are fatty acids found in coconut and palm kernel oil. MCT oil is a convenient supplement that adds fatty acids to your diet without altering your routine. Some of the benefits of MCT oil are weight loss, muscle recovery, mental health improvement and it can also help prevent Alzheimer's and dementia. MCT oil is most commonly enjoyed in bulletproof coffee, but can even be enjoyed in smoothies or even salad dressings.

In this guide, we will review different MCT oils so that you can find your perfect fit!

Alpha Health – MCT Oil

Alpha Health's MCT Oil is a medium concentration. This is the most commonly used MCT oil. Alpha's MCT oil is 100% pure, composed of 60% caprilic acid and 40%

capric acid. This MCT oil caters to individuals who are interested in weight loss and bodybuilding or if you're looking to prevent degenerative diseases such as Alzheimer's. Overall, this medium concentration MCT oil satisfies the body's need for good fats and nutrients without being stored as fat. Enjoy this MCT oil in a bulletproof coffee to start your day energized and focused!

• Fuels the body and brain

• Easily metabolized in the liver and converted into energy

• 100% pure, composed of 60% caprillic acid and 40% capric acid

• Great supplement for individuals interested in weight loss and body building

Bulletproof – Brain Octane MCT Oil

Bulletproofs Brain Octane MCT Oil is a MCT oil with high concentration. Bulletproofs MCT oil can help individuals reach their peak performance all day – especially with demanding tasks or during intermittent fasting. Bulletproofs MCT Oil should be used as part of a ketogenic or low carb diet. The suggested serving is using 1 teaspoon per day and slowly increasing the dosage. Avoid taking on an empty stomach, as it may result in a stomach ache. This product can be used in C, smoothies, and salad dressings.

• Supports energy metabolism at the cellular level

• Quickly and easily absorbed by the body, and not stored as far

• Does not increase cholesterol

• Rebalances the yeast in the gut

Nutiva – Organic MCT Powder

MCT is most commonly in an oil form, but Nutiva offers this popular supplement in a powder form. MCT powder is a creamy alternative to oil – it blends beautifully into beverages and is gentler on the digestive system. This MCT powder still remains low-carb diet and ketogenic friendly because there are zero net carbs. Overall, this product keeps your gut happy and healthy while providing you with the benefits of MCT.

• Delivers digestible fatty acids that quickly convert to ketones

• A great alternative to MCT oil

• 3g of fibre from prebiotic acacia fibre

• Suggested serving is one 10g scoop

St.Francis – MCT Liquid Coconut Oil

St.Francis offers a coconut oil with MCT combined. The liquid coconut oil's main purpose is to be used as a culinary cooking oil. If you want to use the product for medicinal purposes – 5 tbsp. per day is recommended. It can be taken alone or mixed with other foods. This coconut oil stays liquid and non-rancid at room temperature and is in a convenient and easy to use pourable form. Overall, this product is great for individuals who are looking for the benefits of coconut oil / MCT oil in a casual and convenient form.

• Provides a healthful combination of coconut oil and medium chain triglycerides (MCT)

• Assists the body in fending off viruses, and bacteria

• A heart-healthy superfood that helps prevent cardiovascular problems

• A natural antioxidant

Overall, MCT oil is a great supplement with a variety of health benefits. Weight loss, preventing cardiovascular problems, provides energy, prevents Alzheimer's and degenerative diseases, and is a natural antioxidant just to name a few! At Goodness Me! We have a variety of MCT oilsthat will work to improve your meal planning by making it convenient to incorporate those healthy fatty acids into your diet.

Conclusion

There's a lot about the brain that doctors and scientists still don't completely understand. However, they're learning more each day. There are still a lot of interesting things to be learned about the part of you that does the most work. Just like the rest of your body, the brain needs a healthy diet, exercise, and the right amount of sleep to perform its best.

Made in the
USA
Middletown, DE